Rope Skipping for Beginners

- The practice book -

How to learn rope jumping quickly,
acquire jumping techniques in no
time and continuously improve your
new skills

Katja Eden

CONTENT

What you can expect in this book

At the thought of jumping rope, some of you will certainly remember the school breaks back then in the playground at elementary school. And surely you are smiling about it now. It was a pastime as a kid, it was fun, and it was literally child's play. Is it still that way today?

Who would have thought that "rope skipping" would become a recognized sport in which even international competitions are now held.

What has spilled over to Europe as a trend from abroad is also gaining enthusiasm on our doorstep in all age groups and sports groups.

Few other sports require as little and space-saving equipment as rope skipping. So it can be done almost anywhere in the world. Sport shoes, unpack the rope and off you go. It doesn't matter if you are in a hotel room on the other side of the world or simply lack the motivation to go to the gym.

The positive aspects for the cardiovascular system and coordination are definitely not to be ignored. Not only recreational athletes have discovered them, you will also see athletes jumping in professional sports, for example boxers during warm-up, conditioning or coordination training.

The sport offers various opportunities to work out both as a team player and as an individual fighter. Especially for children and teenagers this social aspect is very valuable. On the one hand, you can improve group dynamics as a team, solve problems together or be creative, and on the other hand, there are disciplines where you can measure each other's endurance and speed. This competitive character can also be motivating.

Whether you are a beginner, advanced, competitive, show or recreational group, the most important thing is to never lose the fun and enjoyment of it. As a member of the club, many groups go to the gymnastics festivals that take place regularly. And here, too, there is something for everyone. Whether it's a children's, state, German or international gymnastics festival, there's certainly no chance of boredom.

Of course, you don't want to get bored in this book either, so there's a do-it-yourself chapter that explains simple jumps to copy.

So what are you waiting for? If you're now interested in learning more about this sport, and especially want to give it a try, jump over to the first chapter with gusto.

On the ropes, ready, go.

Trend sport or tradition - The history of the sport

Exactly how and where rope skipping originated is still not known for certain. In the World Wide Web can be found many conjectures and vague claims that put forward different beginnings of the sport, whether geographical or temporal.

According to the most common statements, the sport probably developed over many years from a children's game, or rather a children's activity. Apparently, the sport was brought from Holland to

North America in the 16th or 17th century and then came back to Europe in the 20th century as rope skipping. What is clear, however, is that the first scientific research into the positive aspects that rope skipping has on the cardiovascular system was carried out in the USA at the end of the 1960s.

As a result, the "Jump Rope for Heart" campaign was started in 1978 to promote more regular exercise through jumping rope to show the positive aspects of exercise on the cardiovascular system. This campaign was born in the concern of the "American Heart Association" (AHA).

In the USA, the skipping rope has become an indispensable training tool, which is also available in gyms, and more and more rope skipping courses are also offered in gyms.

The sport has not yet developed quite that far in Germany. Many people don't even know rope skipping as a sport or simply can't imagine it.

The first world championships of Rope Skipping took place in 1996 in Australia.

In the 80s, rope skipping came to Germany through various student exchange programs. Here, unfortunately, it was somewhat lost for the first decade, not belonging to any major club and not officially subordinated or grouped. A lot of preliminary work was necessary for recognition. Training programs, coach education, competition rules and much more were developed.

In the meantime, the course has been set for us as well, because for a few years now, rope skipping has officially become part of the German Gymnastics Federation, and more and more clubs are offering this sport for the first time, because they, too, have become enthusiastic about this sport.

But, now briefly to the name of the sport. In Germany, it is known as rope skipping. Translated, one could comparatively also say rope skipping. This term comes from Canadian transmissions. In the USA, however, the sport is called "Jump Rope" or the activity of jumping rope is called "Rope Jumping" there, which is why a lot of information on the Internet can be found not only under the European known Rope Skipping, but also under Jump Rope and Rope Jumping. No matter what it is called, the main thing is that it is fun.

Prevention, health and fitness

Jumping rope is the perfect endurance workout. From the outside it may seem like a lower-body workout, but anyone who has tried it for themselves will notice how out of breath you get after just a few minutes of jumping. Depending on the intensity of the workout, you will later feel the strain on large muscle groups of the lower as well as the upper extremities, i.e. arms and legs. In the upper body, mainly the shoulder area and arms are used. In the lower body, thigh, calf and foot muscles. By using these several large muscle groups, rope skipping becomes an endurance sport, which can be adapted in its intensity to every person and every form of the day due to the many variable parameters. The faster you jump, the more intensively your cardiovascular system has to work, which is the basis of good endurance training. By exercising regularly for 20 to a maximum of 30 minutes for about three to five times a week, you can reduce the risk of various cardiovascular diseases such as high blood pressure, heart attack and stroke, or other diseases such as diabetes and osteoporosis, as well as reduce the risk of cancer.

Not only the cardiovascular system and your endurance benefit from this ingenious sport, but also your coordination, speed, agility and strength.

The main focus of the training is certainly on endurance. Rope skipping is simply a super endurance sport. The intensity can be well adjusted by different parameters (as described in the chapter Jumping Techniques). Not only the speed directly influences the intensity, but also the type of jump and how much muscle mass is active.

Rope skipping also puts a lot of strain on coordination. The coordination of arms and legs alone is already a challenge for beginners during the basic jump.

In addition, there are always ways to make the jump even more complicated and coordinatively challenging. If a jump becomes too easy or monotonous for you, jump it forward, backward, at a different speed, or even more difficult, in double under.

Several figures have to be executed to the music with well-tuned hand-foot coordination and additionally with the appropriate timing of the rope and a good sense of time. In the process, one or the other time not only a knot is created in the rope, but also in your arms or even in your thoughts. The old saying "practice makes perfect" is apt here. Often it makes more sense not to pay too much attention to the execution, but to let your thoughts run free and just jump on it.

If you have found the usual balance training too dry, you have also found a solution here. Rope skipping also promotes balance, especially if single-leg jumps are integrated into your training.

Of course, the speed is mainly promoted at very fast speeds of the ropes. In this training area are usually only competitive or professional athletes.

Also train or challenge some figures in the area of agility. One of the reasons why the Rope Skipping belongs to the German Gymnastics Federation. Some gymnastic elements can also be performed in the rope, which are rather intended for advanced gymnasts. For the flexibility and thus the execution of certain jumps, stretching within the training sessions is inevitable, otherwise the risk of injury can increase significantly.

Rope skipping is definitely not a strength training that promotes strong muscle building. Nevertheless, strength can also be improved during training. The leg strength is used the most, which can also be increased by the jumps. For example, an easy jump does not strain the leg muscles as much as a double or triple under does. Increased upper body training plays an important role in gymnastics jumps. Also, a rope that has integrated weights increases the training effect of the upper body. In addition, the torso must perform special holding work, especially during asymmetrical exercises, for example, also during a knee up, and is automatically trained during such jumps.

Also a big plus of the sport is that there is generally a very low risk of injury in rope skipping, especially after sufficient warm-up. In contrast to classic jogging, it is easier on the joints of the knees and ankles because the jumps are cushioned on the forefoot. In the classic jogging of recreational athletes without forefoot running, the heel as the first contact with the ground puts significantly more pressure on the knees and hip joints.

If you don't want to do rope skipping as your only workout, you can, for example, incorporate skipping sessions into your HIIT (high-intensity interval training) or circuit training (see chapter Do-it-yourself / workout suggestions)

Not to mention the positive effects on your mind. Exercise releases endorphins and makes us happy. Do you know the feeling of that inner, deepest satisfaction when you've pushed through your sports program? After all, there are no excuses when jumping rope such as "the way to the gym is too long" or the like. You can unpack your rope anywhere, whether at home, in your hotel room, or on a jog, and jump for it.

Team player or
lone wolf

In Rope Skipping you will get your money's worth as a team player and as an individual.

There are jumps as pairs, such as the mill ("Wheel"). Here each jumper has one end of the rope of himself and the other end of the rope of the partner in his hand. The ropes beat alternately in the same direction at a steady pace, which looks like a mill from the side. Another way to jump as a pair is called pair interaction. Here the partners either have a rope in pairs and this is also swung by both or only one partner has the rope and jumps around the other partner without the rope. If you don't have enough imagination, you can enter the names of the jumps in the internet and you will surely find some amazing videos. Also on many of today's popular media platforms can be found numerous videos on the subject of rope skipping and jump rope.

If more jumpers are available, you can jump Double Dutch, for example. For this you need to be at least three - divided into two swingers and one jumper.

With a jumper count of five or more, you can create a box of ropes or a Rainbow with three or four different sizes of rope all swinging into each other to resemble a rainbow.

As a single jumper, the jumps can be increased from the simplest basic jumps to the infinite of the degree of difficulty and speed. And when no jump is too complicated, you invent a new one yourself. Also, using different ropes can make some jumps easier to perform.

A prime example is the classic competitive disciplines, which are partly about speed and partly about creativity, as well as the level of difficulty.

Rope Skipping as a competitive sport

In Germany, too, there are now competitions in the field of rope skipping.

These are divided, as in the rest of the gymnastics areas, first of all into genders and of course into individual or group competitions and in detail into age groups. In some cases, they are additionally divided into difficulty levels.

In individual competitions, "speed" is considered one of the typical disciplines. In this, the jumper looks as if he is running on the spot. The knees are pulled forward towards the chest alternately and the rope must be passed under each foot. The judges, who act as referees in the competition, always count the contact of the right foot with the ground. The jumps completed within the allotted time are then documented. The usual time limits are 30 seconds, 60 seconds and 120 seconds.

In the following section I have listed a few competition results and world records in Rope Skipping.

Joey Motsay jumped rope for a total of 33 hours and 20 minutes without a break in 2009. You think of that again when you take a soothing break after 10 minutes of jumping at a stretch, completely out of breath and sweaty, simply incredible.

In 30 seconds Single Rope Double under very good jumpers jump between 70 and 90 jumps.

Approximately 70 to 95 jumps can be performed in 30 seconds of speed.

Approximately 350 to 440 jumps are possible within 180 seconds of speed.

The above data were all documented from German competitions. Of course, the figures still differ between men and women.

A Chinese jumper achieved the world record in 2015 with 108 jumps in 30 seconds.

The Double Under competition is also timed. The jumper swings the rope under his feet twice within one jump phase. This process counts as one jump. Usually this jump is performed for 30 seconds. Again, the judges count and document the number.

Freestyle, which is also a characteristic part of the individual competitions, requires the most creativity. Each participant prepares his or her own freestyle in training, preferably weeks before the competition, selects music for it and performs it as flawlessly as possible on the day of the competition. Here, too, certain requirements must be met, such as the duration of the routine, and a given area must be filled with the selected jumps.
During the competitions, a track adapted to the start signal is played. There is a specific track for each discipline that is jumped for time. These can also be played on the website of the German Gymnastics Federation (Deutscher Turner-Bund e. V.: Speed-Tracks (dtb.de)).

The announcements of the competitions on district and state level can be seen on the homepages of the respective gymnastics federation, the dates of the world championship can be found on the homepage of the German Gymnastics Federation. There are also specifications and guidelines for registration and qualification.

Recreational sports, show groups, camps and gymnastics festivals

Rope skipping is a wonderful recreational sport. There is no age limit for this sport. Anyone who enjoys it can practice it.

Meanwhile, it is offered in several sports clubs. In clubs there are most often groups for children and teenagers. Rope skipping can be offered to children from about 5 years of age. Again, it is not the age or height of the jumper that matters, but rather the level of difficulty that can be jumped. This way, advanced jumpers can practice more difficult figures and beginners can consolidate the basics. On the other hand, a mixed group can benefit greatly from each other. This is a good social aspect to offer mixed groups for children. The advanced players help the beginners, who can learn from the advanced players. Both sides benefit from a mixed group. In addition, you become creative together and create new figures, jumps and choreographies, because for certain combinations or figures, small, light children or large, stronger young people are an advantage.

Mixed groups of beginners and advanced are also useful for show groups. The children are naturally pleased to be able to perform the jumps and sequences they have learned, and each of them is proud of what they have learned and can show. Therefore, it makes sense to give even the "beginners" space in performances. Of course, the buildup from easy to complex of jumps and choreography also makes sense during performances and shows. This way the audience can see how the beginnings are and how the jumps can be increased more and more.

An important part of the show is certainly the music. It makes a completely different impression when the music matches the jumps and the action on stage with every beat. When it gets quieter, the ropes on stage should also be jumped a little slower and calmer or even not jumped at all. For an intermediate part the non-jumping techniques are especially suitable (see chapter Do-it-yourself). If the music is loud and dominant, the ropes should also be "the place to be". What really makes the decisive impression at shows are the transitions that are supposed to lead from choreography to choreography. Often the rope changes of the jumpers represent a small "interruption" or "disturbance", which must be bridged well, so that the spectator always has something to see somewhere on the stage, which captivates him, in order to let the rope changes of the remaining jumpers at the other end of the stage move into the shade.

Likewise, it is nice to show the complete range of this great sport during performances. From single jumps to synchronized choreographies, pair jumps and group choreographies.

To improve group cohesion, you can participate in rope skipping camps and gymnastics festivals as a competitive, show and recreational group.

Rope skipping camps are quite typical for this sport, which was probably also transferred from America to us.

A camp could look like this, for example: The registered groups of a state gymnastics association meet for four to five days to train with each other, learn from each other, have fun and somehow get through the announced sore muscles.

Accommodation can usually be provided in schools. The classrooms are the dormitories, there are showers, toilets and optimally a dining area, cafeteria or similar.

Over the duration of the camp, there is a tight training schedule, which gives one or the other already on the second day strong muscle soreness. Not only do you get to know many new like-minded people, but you also learn new jumps and figures.

At the conclusion of the camp, a camp show can be presented to parents, friends and interested parties where everyone can show what new things they have learned.

Usually, a so-called cam routine is also practiced over the training days, in which all participants learn the same jump sequence and perform it as synchronously as possible at the end. For this, everyone gets the same T-shirts, which the jumpers get to keep and should remind them for a long time of the great, but also very exhausting time.

Back at home in the club, the jumpers who participated in the camp can show and teach the newly learned jumps and tricks to those who stayed at home. In this way, the skills are automatically passed on and the motivation is rekindled again and again.

The gymnastics festivals are organized by the state associations and require long-term and sophisticated organization, because when around 5,000 gymnasts storm the host city over a weekend, every detail has to be planned. It would not be the first time that the trains are overcrowded or that the shower water gets so cold towards the end that one is surprised that no ice cubes tumble out of the pipe yet. But it is also precisely these experiences that make the gymnastics festivals.

There are alternating state children's and state gymnastics festivals, as well as the German or even International Gymnastics Festival. Here, the full range of movement is offered for all participants and there is certainly something suitable for everyone.

Groups can apply to be show groups, participate in workshops, sign up for competitions or take part in fun competitions. Of course, at every gymnastics festival there is a specially devised choreography as the "gymnastics festival dance". This is danced again and again in between and it is simply an unbelievable feeling when a huge amount of children, young people and of course also helpers and coaches "put on a flash mob".

All day long there are sports activities on the sports grounds and in the evening the day ends with a party. On one of the evenings, the city in which the next state children's or state gymnastics festival will be held presents itself. These two are held in alternation.

Accommodation for the many participants is distributed among the schools of the city. Often, several clubs share a classroom. So you quickly get to know many other sports-mad children, young people and coaches. The gymnastics festival evenings and sometimes even nights are truly legendary. You simply have to experience it for yourself.

The clubs usually remember this special time fondly for a long time to come.

From theory to practice

EQUIPMENT

The equipment includes, first and foremost, the rope. But there is not only one rope, but many different ropes made of different materials, which accordingly also bring different properties.

The **Speed Rope** is a rope made of plastic. It is about half as heavy as the Beaded Rope and should be able to rotate freely in the handle when jumping. High speeds can be trained well with this rope. Another quality test is that it should not stretch more than 2 cm at most when pulled. Generally, it is good if it feels rather firm.

This rope is available with standard handles or extended handles, which are especially useful for "criss-cross" variations, as these are intended to serve as an extension of the arms. The rope with extended handles is called Long Handle.

The **High Speed Rope** and the **Wire Rope** are essentially for competitions. Some of the ropes consist of an inner part, which is made of wire, and an outer part made of plastic, which sheathes the inner one. The best ropes are those with ball bearings, as they offer the least risk of twisting and thus wasting valuable time, especially when competing.

The High Speed and Wire Ropes can become incredibly fast due to their low weight and are therefore not suitable for beginners or untrained people. The more the competitors benefit from it, because they have less load respectively have to use less strength in the upper body.

The **Beaded Rope** is a rope with many short, hard plastic pieces, which keeps it from twisting. When it hits the ground while jumping, it is much louder than the Speed Rope. The rope itself is heavier, which makes it easier to perform slow jumps and still produce a nice arc shape. Also, this rope is used in Pair interaction and Wheel. Often the plastic particles are in bright colors, so the ropes have a great wow effect on the audience during performances.

Likewise, there are ropes to focus the training effect of the upper body, which contain integrated weights. It is possible to distinguish ropes with weights exclusively in the handles from ropes with complete weight in the rope itself. In order to give the upper body a stronger but balanced workout, the rope with the distributed weights is recommended.

There are also woven ropes, which are usually made of synthetic material. The biggest advantage is that these do not hurt when you get them off. Unfortunately, however, they are not optimal for swinging, because the swing from the wrists is not enough and therefore requires more strength again. Mostly, the woven ropes are therefore rather used as a long rope or for the Double Dutch, in which then, for example, a third person jumps.

The rope length for a single jumper can be specifically measured as follows: Holding the rope by the handles, one handle in the right hand, the other in the left hand, climb with both feet on the rope, which is then stretched toward the armpits. The ends of the handles should almost touch the armpits, but not go beyond them.

Speed Ropes are always made a little shorter than the "formula" above, because the body position is slightly bent during speed and a shorter rope means at the same time less effort at higher speed.

When buying it is important to pay attention to the fact that the ropes are fixed in the handle with a small extra tube and a needle (similar to a staple). This allows you to shorten the rope as desired and fix it again, without neglecting the good rotating property in the handle.

With the Beaded Ropes, simply untie the knot in the handle and any number of small plastic pieces can be threaded out or on until the length fits perfectly.

The handles are usually also made of plastic. The surfaces can be smooth, slightly ribbed or somewhat rough. If you need more grip, you can wrap the plastic handles with tape. In addition to the "normal" handles, there are also extra long handles called "Long Handle", as already briefly mentioned with the Speed Ropes. These are especially helpful for many cross jump variations, as they lengthen the jumper's arm. Nevertheless, it is a completely different feeling when jumping and jumps usually have to be practiced thoroughly again with the long handle, even if they were already well implemented with usual handles.

Actually, you can train with the rope almost everywhere, but only almost. There are more suitable surfaces such as, of course, the gym floor, which is super suitable, or even carpet, if it is not too soft. If you train frequently on very hard surfaces such as stone or asphalt, the joints can be much more stressed and strained. In addition, this surface damages the ropes in the long run. They become very rough and wear out visibly.

Any clothing is suitable. The best is usually relatively body-hugging, tight clothing, so that it does not get caught in the rope.

It is highly recommended to wear good sports shoes that have cushioning on the forefoot and provide good stability to the foot.

JUMP AND SWING TECHNIQUE

Jumping technique is crucial in rope skipping. However, the body position is not the same for all jumps, but this will be discussed in the course of the text. The feet always have contact with the ground only with the forefoot. This means that the jump can sometimes be initiated by bending the knees and then be cushioned again when the feet hit the ground. Almost never does the whole foot touch the ground between two jumps. Doing so would cause you to lose momentum. The first contact with the ground is made exclusively with the ball of the foot. From there, the foot can be rolled off. Sometimes you can even hear an incorrect jumping technique, because those who jump correctly are barely audible. On the other hand, someone who lands with the entire foot, for example, sounds like a trampling animal. A suitable floor that is somewhat springy, such as is found in most gymnasiums, also contributes to the correct jumping technique. A slightly springy floor also helps the rope to glide across the floor rather than bouncing off the ground.

To save forces, it is important to jump only a few centimeters high, because it must just be able to slide the rope under your feet. If you jump too high in the long run, you lose an incredible amount of strength and waste your energy. However, if you jump double and triple under, you will notice that you actually have to jump higher there than in the basic jumps, for example.

To save strength, you can jump the so-called jog step. This involves jumping from one leg to the other, which automatically results in a small right/left movement. The second leg always supports with a short contact to the ground, but takes over almost no body weight.

The swinging motion in Speed Rope comes mainly from the wrist. The upper arms should remain as close to the body as possible so that the rope can form a symmetrical, even arc shape above the head. After training speed may well be that your forearms "burn" and the next day there will also be noticeable muscle soreness.

When swinging the Long Rope or Double Dutch, the movement should be performed larger and comes from the entire arm, because especially when performing jumps from Gymnastics, the swingers are required to adapt to the pace of the jumper and the size of the movement.

The entire body posture is upright for "normal" jumps, and also tends to be a little more bent over for certain figures. Especially with speed, it is important to make yourself a little smaller, as shorter ropes tend to be used here, primarily to save energy and power. The knees are then pulled forward upwards towards the chest as quickly as possible.

MUSIC SELECTION

The choice of music can be crucial in rope skipping for the wow effect of the audience. The very first thing that would be important is that the beat is easy to hear and has a comfortable speed for jumping, because even by jumping extremely slowly you waste an incredible amount of energy. The best range is between 125 and 150 bpm. Most equipment these days also has a slider to adjust the speed. So you can well try out in which range it is most comfortable for you to jump.

So much can be expressed with the help of music. It makes movements bigger, more powerful and amplifies emotions.

The sense of rhythm is also particularly challenging for some people and may require some practice at first.

Do-it-yourself

Before starting the first simple jumps, warming up the entire body is very important. This will reduce the risk of injury, as mentioned in the chapter Prevention, Health and Fitness.

First, the entire body should be warmed up a little by, for example, light jogging or fast walking, which is easier on the joints. Otherwise, movements and variations in walking can serve as a warm-up. To do this, you can walk quickly forward, backward and sideways. If you like, do side gallops, alternately pulling your knees way up and then your heels toward your butt. The exercises can be done well both while walking and running.

After that, the different muscle groups are warmed up even more specifically.

While standing, push up on your toes and slowly sink back down to the floor with your heel.

Furthermore, you can perform classic squats and finally combine both exercises. The hips can be rotated alternately in both directions. Lunges can also serve well as a warm-up exercise.

During the exercises, always ensure proper execution.

For the arms, first circle both arms forward alternately and change direction after several circles. It is also essential to warm up the wrists by "circling" them.

Not only warming up is important, but also special stabilization units for the ankles, for example, are essential.

For this, practice the one-leg stand in all possible variations. You can also practice this every day while brushing your teeth. The best thing to do is to make a movement in the air with your raised foot, such as a lying figure eight or your own name. Changing the support surface, such as standing on soft mats, on the sofa or on an air cushion, also makes the exercise more difficult and makes the foot or the foot and lower leg muscles work in a complex way. In fact, by wearing shoes all the time and walking on flat asphalt, our feet unlearn their original function, flexibility and strength over time.

Unlike stabilization exercises, depending on the jumps being trained, only dynamic springy stretching should be done before the training session to maintain tension in the muscle. However, anyone who integrates gymnastics into their training must be careful to stretch extensively to avoid risking a strain.

For a beginner's workout, it's enough to squeeze in a short stretching session.
For this, you can take your arms up while standing and simply stretch upwards with alternating arms.

Also while standing, open both arms to the side and pull them back as far as possible. The head remains upright. Then do the same exercise with a different arm position. The arms form a diagonal, i.e. one arm stretches upwards to the right and the other downwards to the left, for example. Then switch again.

Also very important is the stretching of the hand flexors and extensors.

To do this, extend one arm forward and fold the hand in toward the palm or back of the hand. The other hand helps here to get into the maximum possible flexion or extension.

On the legs, the calves should be dynamically stretched by walking forward with a lunge. The front leg is bent, the back leg is extended and the heel touches the floor. If no stretch is felt in the rear calf, the lunge should be increased. Again, the stretch is springy, meaning the heel touches the floor and then is lifted back off the floor a little by rolling over the forefoot.

The more detailed description of the stretches are in the subchapter Training suggestions in the Cool-down section.

As mentioned above, these stretches should not be held statically and to the maximum before a beginner workout, but dynamically and springily. That is, you always move a little more towards the maximum position and then give back a little, without holding the maximum position for a long time.

With the following non-jumping techniques we slowly approach the handling with the rope. These are especially suitable for beginners or can be well integrated into a freestyle.

In principle, the name of this jump group is self-explanatory. They are "jumps" that do not require jumping over the rope.

In the **Windmill,** both handles of the rope are held in one hand. The rope swings either on the side of the hand that has both handles or on the opposite side, which can also be done alternately.

If the Windmill is integrated into a freestyle routine, this is usually called a **Side Swing** when performed once.

Other techniques are the **wraps**. You can do arm wraps and leg wraps. The rope is swung forward and wrapped around an arm or leg, unwound and swung further. Continuing to swing can also be used as a change of direction. So if you wind the rope forward after a jump, it will automatically come from the front to the back after unwinding, which would mean you continue jumping backward.

Other **non-jumping** techniques are **releases**. A rope end is released or thrown from various initial positions and then caught again. This technique can be directly surrounded by jumps, which can look very spectacular. However, it also comes with a risk, because no matter how many times you've practiced releases, if you get excited during a performance and then fail to catch the end of the rope, it somehow interrupts the flow while jumping.

To approach the jumps, you can practice the **Step Through.**

Here the rope is held normally, so each handle in his hand. One arm is held more at head height, the other at crotch height. You get in with one leg on one side, so to speak, and the rope swings around you at the back so that you can get out again on the other side. If you feel confident doing this, you can turn around yourself in the meantime, either a 180° turn or directly a 360° turn.

JUMPING TECHNIQUES

Now we come to the first jumps.

The easiest jumps are the Easy Jump and the Double Bounce.

In **Easy Jump,** you jump over the rope each time, which tends to have a faster speed, but it can also be increased as you go, so you still have the option to start slow.

The **Double Bounce** includes a so-called intermediate jump, where the rope does not pass under the feet. It tends to be much slower than an Easy Jump and since momentum is otherwise lost in the long pause, an intermediate bounce is included.

The **jog-step** is a strength-saving jump that I have already taken up in the subchapter Jump and Swing Technique. You jump from one leg to the other, with the second leg always supporting the ground.

With the **Foot Catch,** you can stop the rope specifically. If several jumpers do this at the same time, this "jump" alone looks really great.

Of course, all three presented basic jumps can also be jumped backwards. As a first simple sequence of jumps you can connect the three basic jumps, which is not so easy for the beginning because of the change of speed.

These were the most important basics, now follow some leg combinations.

One of the simplest leg combinations is the "**jumping jack**", also called **side straddle.** Surely you already know this jump without the rope. The arms swing the rope further and the legs open sideways and close again. With each swing of the rope the legs open and close. An extension of this jump is the **X-it**. Here the legs, after they have been opened in the jumping jack, are not only brought to each other when closing, but even crossed.

The next jump **Straddle forward**, which is also known as jumping jack back-and-forth, works similarly. The difference is that the legs open alternately forward and backward and close again in the middle.

For example, a related jump, the **Heel Tap,** involves moving only one foot forward and tapping the heel on the ground, pulling back in, performing an Easy Jump, and switching sides.

If the heel has no contact with the ground in front and the foot is only kicked forward, the jump is obviously called a **kick.**

In **skiing,** sometimes called **slalom**, the jumper imagines he is standing on a line and then jumps with both legs once to the right and the next time to the left of the line. With each jump, the rope is passed under the feet.

The **twist** most closely resembles the slalom/ski. However, the jumper keeps both feet constantly in the center and rotates the lower body to the right and left so that the tips of the feet point alternately to the right and left.

The **knee up** is also often part of choreos. To do this, you alternately pull one knee toward your chest while jumping, set the leg back down and switch sides. Again, an action takes place with each rope turn, which means knee up, jump together once, and other knee up. While one knee is tucked, you are practically jumping on one leg. Knee up can be jumped fast and slow, with the fast version being much easier.

If the jump knee up is combined with a kind of kick (leg should be kicked higher than in the kick described above), the so-called can is created, which actually reminds of the Funkenmariechen in the Cologne carnival. Between the two jumps, the foot taps the floor once in the middle, but does not take any body weight.

The next jump is called a **boxer**. It is again a kind of single leg jump, but this time the lifted leg is not bent forward, but the knee is bent backwards at a 90° angle. So you jump over the rope 2 times and this is counted as one boxer.

These were the simplest leg combinations in rope skipping.

Continue with arm combinations

The simplest arm combination is the classic **cross**, also called **criss cross.**

To do this, cross your forearms at the level of your belly button. It is important that the handle ends of the rope are visible when you are standing with your back to another person, because only then can the rope form a nice arc around you and you will not get caught. To make this easier, there are the Long Handle Ropes that were introduced in the Equipment topic. You jump once with your arms crossed and open them again. The same jump can of course be done backwards, although this requires a bit more practice.

Similarly, the cross jump can be performed forward while crossing the arms behind the body.

If the Criss Cross is connected with the Side Swing, it is called Side Swing Criss Cross and admittedly looks complicated to spectators. A Side Swing is followed by a Criss Cross and then again by a Side Swing. It is best to change the side of the Side Swing. This makes the sequence even more varied.

You see: There are countless variations and variants that you can try out, practice or invent yourself.

Again a kind of cross is the "**eb**". Here, one arm is crossed in front of the body and the other arm is crossed behind the body. In preparation for the crossing of the arms, a **side swing is** automatically created, which means that the rope swings sideways past the body and theoretically does not have to be jumped over. Nevertheless, it is best to keep jumping in order not to lose the beat on the one hand and the swing on the other. In addition, if this jump becomes part of a choreography, it gives a nicer overall picture if everyone continues jumping synchronously and does not simply stop.

Yet another variation of the classic cross jump is the **toad,** which raises the difficulty level significantly. This time, both arms are crossed in front of the body again, but one arm is crossed under the opposite leg, again creating a kind of single-leg jump, which makes the execution even more difficult. Generally, in the classic cross, it doesn't matter which arm crosses above and below, i.e. which one crosses directly at the belly button and which one crosses away from the body. In the Toad, however, only the arm close to the body can cross under the leg. You should therefore think carefully beforehand about which arm will be close to the body and which leg will then need to be lifted. A good tip is to push the arm crossed under the leg far towards the back of the knee of the lifted leg to make the space in the rope as large as possible, so that there is a greater chance of completing the jump without getting stuck. I also recommend that you practice the jump or swing sequence a few times "dry", i.e. without the rope, before your first attempt. The brain learns the sequence with an increasing number of repetitions and remembers the feeling of the movement, until at some point you no longer have to think about it, but can simply jump off.

If you want to lift the left leg, the right arm must be crossed close to the body, and if you cross under the right leg, the left arm must be positioned close to the body.

Opening this jump seems a bit like jumping forward, as you jump from one leg that was still in contact with the ground to the other leg that was crossed under.

In Inverse Toad, the crossing arm is performed from the outside under the equilateral leg.

Crougar is also performed in arm and leg combination. One arm is passed under the same-sided leg, respectively the leg is lifted and you jump once over the rope in this position. To dissolve the jump, perform a side swing to the opposite side.

For coordination professionals, the last two jumps can be used to create a combination called a "pretzel".

If you mix the different arm and leg combinations, you can create countless jumps. For example, a criss cross with crossed legs or a twist or slalom also with crossed arms is ideal for this. There are no limits to you and your creativity.

Basically, it should be said about all jumps that everyone usually has a "better" side and often you only master the jumps on one side, especially in the beginning. Therefore, it is important to practice all jumps on both sides. It challenges the coordination even more than always being satisfied with the "good" side.

Before you get your hands completely knotted, let's switch to the twists section.

The most frequently performed turn is the 180° turn with swing direction change. It is possible with both the easy jump and the double bounce. After a jump forward, a side swing is initiated, which the body follows through 180°. The rope now swings backwards quite automatically. Here you can initiate another Side Swing after one or more jumps backwards, ideally in the same direction, so that you have made a whole 360° turn in total. Once you have reached the front, you will notice that the rope is now coming from the front again and that you have no choice but to jump forward.

The next jump is a simple basic jump, but due to the speed it becomes a real challenge - **double** and **triple under**. For this, the jumper should jump a little higher than usual, so that the rope can be hit two or three times under the feet. At the same time, the arms must accelerate significantly and the timing for the jump must fit here, so that not too much power is wasted.

Speed is also important in the competition discipline **Speed**, which was described in more detail in the chapter Competitive Sports.

If you have mastered all the above jumps, you can already call yourself advanced.

Let's move on to the partner jumps. There are several variations where a couple use one or two ropes (see chapter Team Player or Individual).

When a rope is used in pairs, it is called **Pair Interaction**. One partner can grab both ends of the rope or each partner can grab one of the rope ends.

For example, if one partner has both ends, he jumps normally on the spot. The other partner jumps into the rope with the jumping partner in front or behind. It is also possible the other way around, so that the jumping partner catches the other. This is possible with the rope running forwards and backwards, as well as from the front and back or with an integrated rotation.

If both partners are leading one end of the rope, both can jump in the same rope at the same time, take turns in what looks like a sort of cross, or one partner is used only as a swinger while the other performs an arm or leg combination or other trick.

Wheel is called a partner exercise where both partners hold one end of their own rope and one end of their partner's rope. You stand next to each other as a couple. The ropes cross in the area between you and behind each of you is basically an arc of rope. The most difficult thing about the Wheel is the staggered use of the two ropes, as one rope points toward the sky while the other hits the ground, so they are always timed in opposite directions. Many different spins, cross jumps and tricks can be practiced in this setting. Wheel with more than 2 jumpers is also possible, for example, you could form a long line.

Now we will go into another section of the jumps. This one is not for beginners, and they are also a challenge for advanced gymnasts. In **gymnastics,** the "kinship" with gymnastics becomes clear.

Essentially, the following three jumps or figures are known, of course there are others, but they are not mentioned here. All three can be performed in single rope as well as in Long Rope or Double Dutch. Targeted and sufficient stretching is very important for the following three jumps.

The **push-up is reminiscent of** a classic push-up. The jumper comes into the squat position, jumps from there into the starting position of a push-up, from there back into the squat position and further into the normal jumping position. With each jump, even into a squat, the rope is passed under the body.

During the **split, the** legs are opened forward and backward similar to a deep lunge or an incomplete split. On the next jump, the legs close back into the squat and you can continue jumping as you wish.

The Frog is reminiscent of a handstand with folded lower legs. These are necessary to get enough momentum for the jump from the hands back to the legs. At every change of position, i.e.

also from the feet to the hands and from the hands to the feet, the rope must be performed under the body.

DoubleDutch jump teams most often. There are two swingers connected by two ropes. Both ropes turn towards the center, that is, the swinger swings from the top to the center and from there to the bottom outside and back up. In it, one person can jump alone or with speed rope, or it is several jumpers combining different jumps or even showing push-up, split or frog. This is part of the master class, because every movement of all participants, as well as the timing with the rope must fit to the point.

A cool-down is also highly recommended after the workout. It slowly shuts down the body, the muscle groups used are stretched in a targeted manner and the training is rounded off overall so that the regeneration of the body is supported.

The most important muscle groups to stretch in the upper body are neck, chest, shoulder and forearm muscles. In the lower body, the hip, thigh and lower leg muscles should be stretched.

The intensity of the training can be adjusted by various parameters. For example, it can be made more intensive by using a faster speed, a higher rope weight, certain demanding jumping techniques and increasing the duration or the number of jumps performed in direct succession.

Less stress can be achieved through increased use of non-jumping techniques, throttled speed and low rope weight.

TRAINING SUGGESTIONS

An exemplary training week with 4 very different training sessions.

Training day 1
20 minutes without warm-up and cool-down
Warm up and light springy stretching
5 minutes jumping in:

– Beginner 30 seconds load / 30 seconds rest

– Advanced 50 sec. load / 10 sec. rest

<u>Jumps in load time:</u>

- Easy jump
- Knee up
- Jumping Jack
- Straddle forward
- Kick

11 minutes of training:

– Beginners see above

– Advanced see above

– Professionals replace the pause times with a jump such as Easy Jump (lower load) or Double under (higher load)

- Easy jump
- Speed
- Easy jump
- Double under
- Easy jump
- Speed
- Easy jump
- Double under
- Easy jump

- Speed
- Easy jump

4 minutes of loose jumping:
– Beginners see above
– Advanced see above

- Jog Step
- Heel Tap
- Kick
- Easy jump

Cool-down with stretching:

Upper body:

Neck muscles: Tilt the head to the side and pull the shoulder down towards the back. It is best to pull the hand towards the back of the hand so that the pull in the neck area is increased.

Chest muscles: Lie on the floor in a supine position and place the legs. The arms are also placed on the floor at the sides at a 90° angle or diagonally (like a Y). The stretch should be felt in the area of the chest muscle.

Shoulder muscles: Do you know the elephant whose trunk you played with your arms as a child? This starting position is well suited for the stretch. However, you don't have to grab your nose here, but your upper arm, so that the stretch arrives at the back of the shoulder.

Forearm muscles: The execution of this stretch has already been touched upon in the Do-it-yourself chapter. One arm is extended forward, the other hand fixes the hand folded towards the palm or back of the hand. Depending on the direction, the wrist flexors or wrist extensors are stretched.

Since the movement of the rope comes from the area of the forearm and wrist, it is important to perform this stretch regularly.

Lower body:

Hip flexors: you go into a big lunge, the front leg on the foot with a right angle at the knee, you can put the back   leg on the knee. The lunge should be large enough that you can feel a stretch pain in the groin area of the back leg. This stretch can be increased by straightening the upper body as well as adding diagonal arm extension.

Front of thigh: It is best to perform the stretch in the lateral position, as this is where there is the least opportunity for evasion. The lower leg is pulled forward toward the chest with the knee bent. The lower hand can fix this position. This should tilt the pelvis backward to increase the stretch in the front of the thigh. The other knee is also bent, the heel is moved towards the buttocks and the lower leg is pulled by the upper hand, which is still free. The stretch should be felt in the front of the thigh (sometimes also in the groin).

Back of thigh: The stretch is possible in standing position or sitting on the floor. While standing, cross your legs and bend forward with your back straight, or while sitting on the floor, also stretch with your back straight toward the tips of your toes, which are tightened to reinforce the stretch.

Calf muscles: The calf muscles can also be stretched with the help of a large lunge. The heel of the back foot must constantly touch the floor. To increase the effect, you can stand on a stair step and push one foot with the heel beyond the step so that the heel can sink down and a significant stretching pain is felt. The knee must remain extended during this process. The other leg takes over the body weight, stands with the entire sole of the foot on the step and is slightly bent at the knee.

<u>Shin muscles</u>: The shin muscles are rarely to be stretched. To do this, place a foot in a standing position without body weight with the back, i.e. the surface of the toes, if possible even with part of the back of the foot. Here you should already be able to feel a slight stretch at the level of the in-step.

Training day 2: HIIT

A HII training is very demanding and stressful for the organism, because in the jumping phases you really have to give 100% for this short training to be effective.

The warm-up can be either jumping, performing exercises or running. Depending on what you are most in the mood for.

In the main part, jumping phases alternate with rest phases. If you have not jumped as a warm-up, it is advisable to first spend two to three minutes getting used to handling the rope again.

After that, the actual training starts.

The load phases, in which jumps are performed, are 30-45 seconds long. For beginners, 30 seconds are suitable, for advanced - 45 seconds.

The rest phases are between 45 seconds and one minute. So if you are aiming for an extra intensive workout, choose the load phase long and the rest phase short, always keeping in mind that you can only give your all during the load phases if you can recover a little in between.

Carry out approximately 6 to 10 load phases.

The cool-down phase is also important after this training in order to reduce the load in a controlled manner.

<u>Training day 3</u>: Speed training
Speed training is very intensive and can be used well as a progress control of one's own performance.

For example, you can time jump certain disciplines every two weeks and document them. This way you can see if you are improving or if your performance is stagnating. Again, sufficient warm-up is the key, and jumping in, where you increase the speed, is also useful.

For beginners are suitable disciplines:

- 30 seconds speed

- 30 seconds easy jump

- 30 seconds criss cross

For advanced students are equally suitable the above disciplines plus:

- 60 and 120 seconds speed

- 30 and 60 seconds Double under

Of course, you can include other disciplines in your progress monitoring.

If you really want to give it your all, I would advise you to train no more than 10 minutes of pure jumping time.

After that, you can always incorporate a few other jumps into your workout, or take it easy. Again, don't forget to finish your workout with the cool-down.

<u>**Training day 4:**</u> **More variety is not possible**

➜ Each exercise is performed only once.

After warming up and jumping in, the 20-minute training session starts. Each jump is performed only once. So today it will be very varied. You can vary the load time as well as the break phase yourself, as explained on the first training day, and find your intensity.

1. easy jump
2. knee up
3. double bounce
4. side swing criss cross
5. boxer
6. jumping jack
7. x-it
8. side swing right/left
9. crougar
10. speed
11. criss cross
12. slalom
13. heel tap
14. easy jump backwards
15. twister
16 Can Can

17. double under

18. kick

19. straddle forward

20. toad

For those who cannot yet perform the more diffi-cult jumps, replace them with another jump.

Also after this part of the workout, finish slowly with loose jumping and the cool-down.

<u>Training Day 5:</u> Repeat Day
For a change, the main part of this training day is not related to a set time, but to the set number of jumps.

After the classic warm-up comes the main part.

Here you could again divide into beginners and advanced. However, I would like to leave some room for your creativity and write down only one training for the beginners in the follow-ing. If you have already been training for a few weeks, you can simply try to complete a higher number of the listed jumps or keep the number but choose a more intensive jump for it.

However, if you do want something to compare to specifically improve and motivate yourself, stop the time it takes you to complete the series of jumps listed below.

- 100   Easy Jump
- 30   Criss Cross
- 30   Knee up
- 30   Jumping Jacks
- 100Speed
- 30Slalom
- 30Boxer
- 30   Twister
- 100Easy   Jump backward
- 20   Can Can
- 100   Speed
- 50   Double Bounce

If you do all the jumps without a break, you will need about 8 minutes for one run. After a sufficient break (about 1 to 2 minutes) you can jump the sequence backwards again or repeat it as often as you like.

After this part of the workout, you should also do some loose jumping and then a cool-down with stretches.

If you can't decide between bodyweight training and rope skipping or if you are looking for a good combination of endurance and strength training, these two training modules can be combined perfectly.

For example, you can warm up with the rope, in the main training part you alternate jumping and exercise phases (with body weight exercises) and in the cool-down you stretch the stressed muscles again as usual.

Here, too, the intensity can be easily regulated via load and pause time.